AF886517

It's easy to get lost in the cancer world

Let NCCN Guidelines for Patients® be your guide

- ✓ Step-by-step guides to the cancer care options likely to have the best results
- ✓ Based on treatment guidelines used by health care providers worldwide
- ✓ Designed to help you discuss cancer treatment with your doctors

National Comprehensive Cancer Network®

NCCN Guidelines for Patients® are developed by the National Comprehensive Cancer Network® (NCCN®)

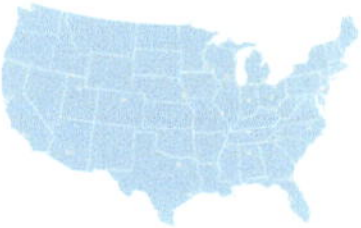

NCCN

- An alliance of leading cancer centers across the United States devoted to patient care, research, and education

Cancer centers that are part of NCCN:
NCCN.org/cancercenters

NCCN Clinical Practice Guidelines in Oncology (NCCN Guidelines®)

- Developed by experts from NCCN cancer centers using the latest research and years of experience
- For providers of cancer care all over the world
- Expert recommendations for cancer screening, diagnosis, and treatment

Free online at
NCCN.org/guidelines

NCCN Guidelines for Patients

- Present information from the NCCN Guidelines in an easy-to-learn format
- For people with cancer and those who support them
- Explain the cancer care options likely to have the best results

Free online at
NCCN.org/patientguidelines

These NCCN Guidelines for Patients are based on the NCCN Guidelines® for Breast Cancer Screening and Diagnosis, Version 1.2022 – June 2, 2022.

NCCN Foundation seeks to support the millions of patients and their families affected by a cancer diagnosis by funding and distributing NCCN Guidelines for Patients. NCCN Foundation is also committed to advancing cancer treatment by funding the nation's promising doctors at the center of innovation in cancer research. For more details and the full library of patient and caregiver resources, visit NCCN.org/patients.

National Comprehensive Cancer Network (NCCN) / NCCN Foundation
3025 Chemical Road, Suite 100
Plymouth Meeting, PA 19462
215.690.0300

NATIONAL COMPREHENSIVE CANCER NETWORK®
NCCN FOUNDATION
Guiding Treatment. Changing Lives.

NCCN Guidelines for Patients are supported by funding from the NCCN Foundation®

To make a gift or learn more, please visit NCCNFoundation.org/donate
or e-mail PatientGuidelines@NCCN.org.

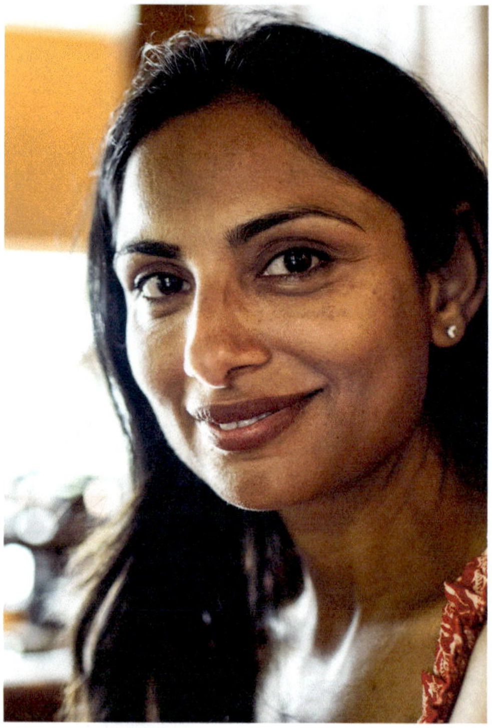
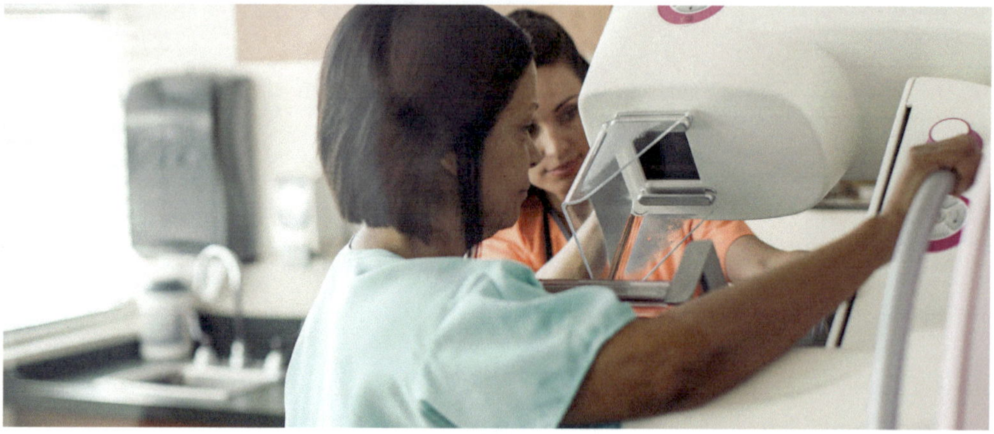
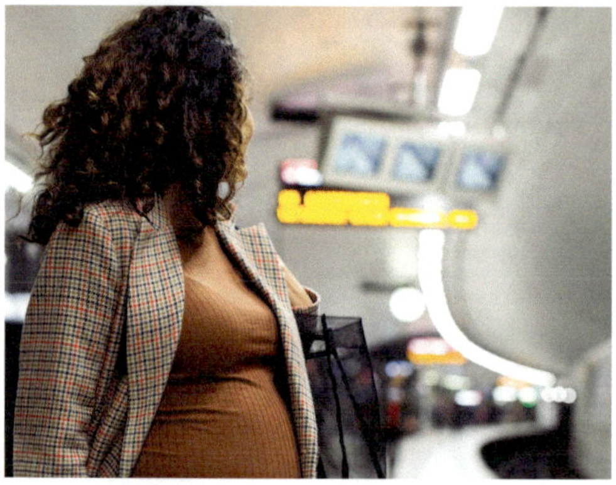
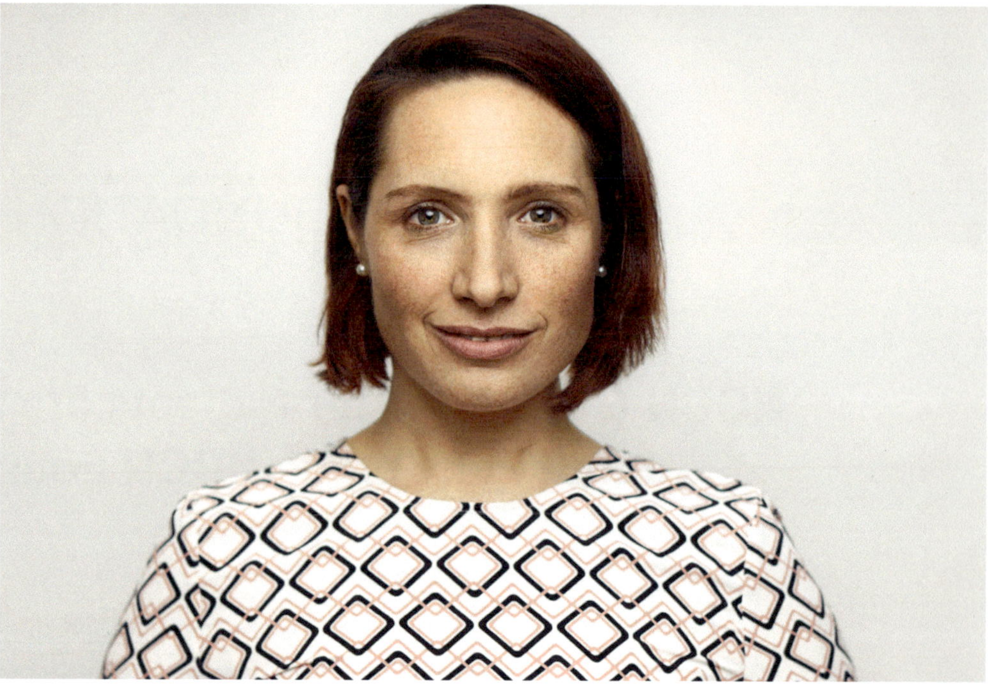
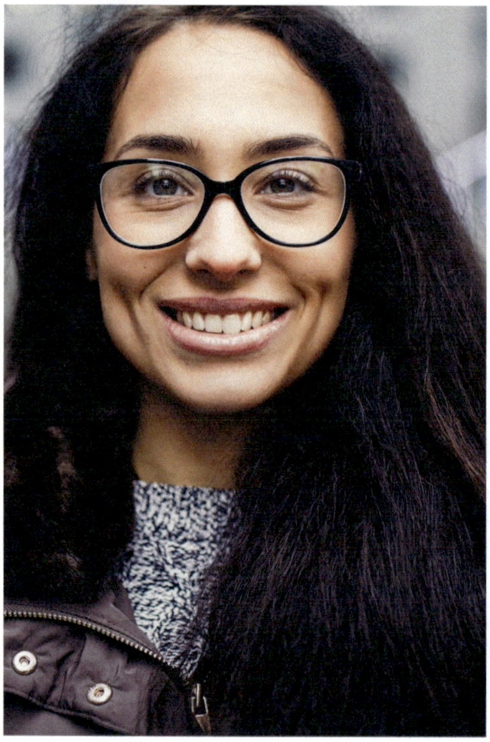
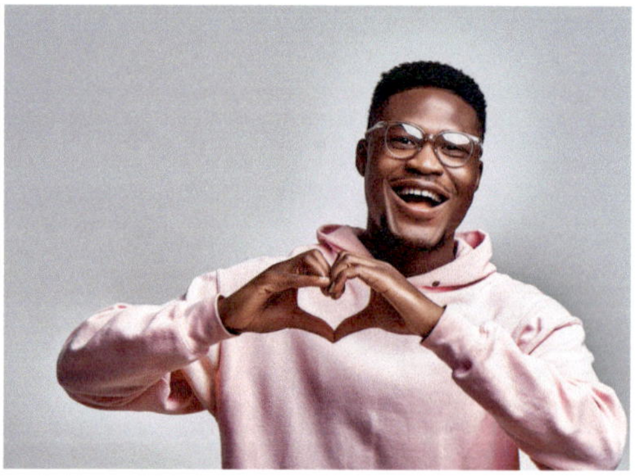
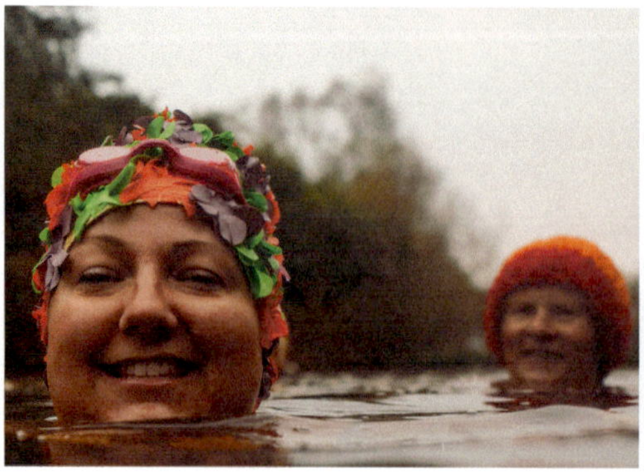
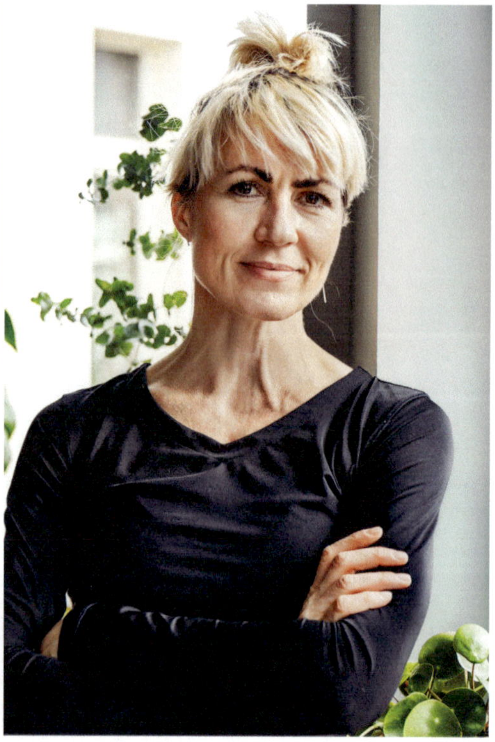

Contents

1
Breast cancer screening basics

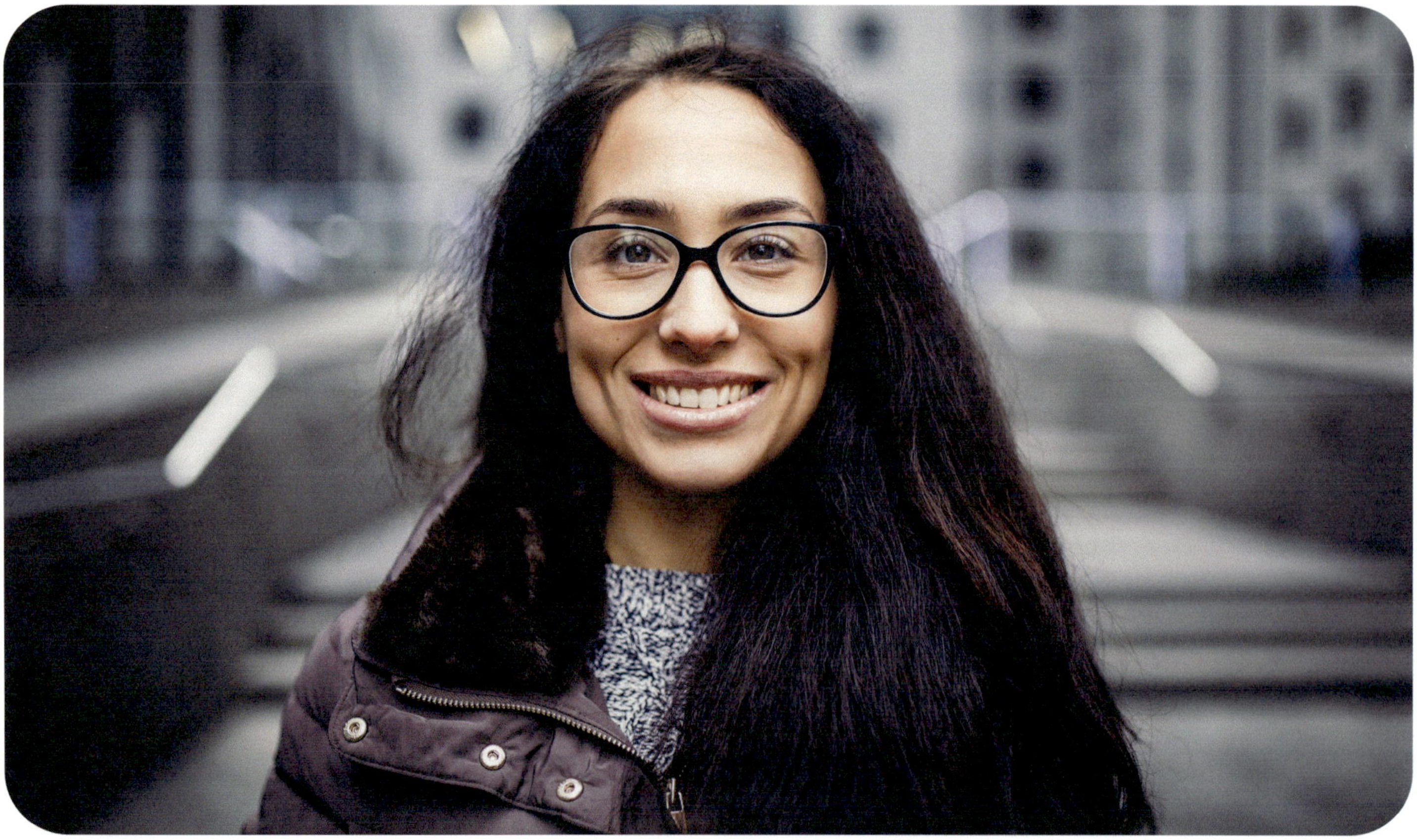

Breast cancer starts in the cells of the breast. Regular screening and breast exams help find breast cancer at its earliest, most treatable stages.

The breast

The breast is an organ and a gland found on the chest. The breast is made of milk ducts, fat, nerves, lymph and blood vessels, ligaments, and other connective tissue. Behind the breast is the pectoral muscle and ribs. Muscle and ligaments help hold the breast in place.

Breast tissue contains glands that can make milk. These milk glands are called lobules. Lobules look like tiny clusters of grapes. Small tubes called ducts connect the lobules to the nipple to carry breast milk.

The ring of darker breast skin is called the areola. The raised tip within the areola is called the nipple. The nipple-areola complex is a term that refers to both parts.

Lymph is a clear fluid that gives cells water and food. It also helps to fight germs or tumor cells. Lymph drains from breast tissue into lymph vessels and travels to lymph nodes near your armpit (axilla). Nodes near the armpit are called axillary lymph nodes (ALNs).

The breast

The breast is a glandular organ made up of milk ducts, fat, nerves, blood and lymph vessels, ligaments, and other connective tissue.

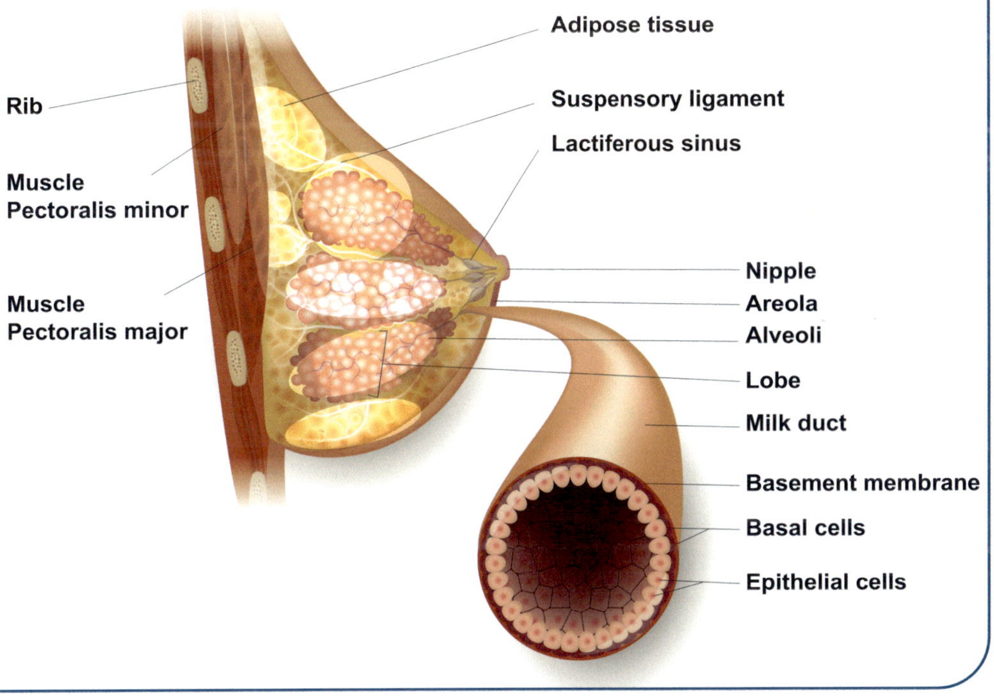

Breast cancer

Breast cancer starts in the cells of the breast. Almost all breast cancers are carcinomas. Carcinomas are cancers that start in the cells that line the inner or outer surfaces of the body.

There are different types of breast carcinoma. The most common types are either ductal or lobular.

- **Ductal carcinoma** starts in the cells that line the milk ducts. Ductal carcinoma is the most common type of breast cancer.
- **Lobular carcinoma** starts in the lobules (milk glands) of the breast.

Anyone can develop breast cancer, including those assigned male at birth. Although there are some differences between those assigned male and those assigned female at birth, treatment is very similar for all genders.

If you are looking for more information on breast cancer, read

- *NCCN Guidelines for Patients: Breast Cancer – Ductal Carcinoma In Situ*, available at NCCN.org/patientguidelines
- *NCCN Guidelines for Patients: Breast Cancer – Invasive*, available at NCCN.org/patientguidelines
- *NCCN Guidelines for Patients: Breast Cancer – Metastatic*, available at NCCN.org/patientguidelines

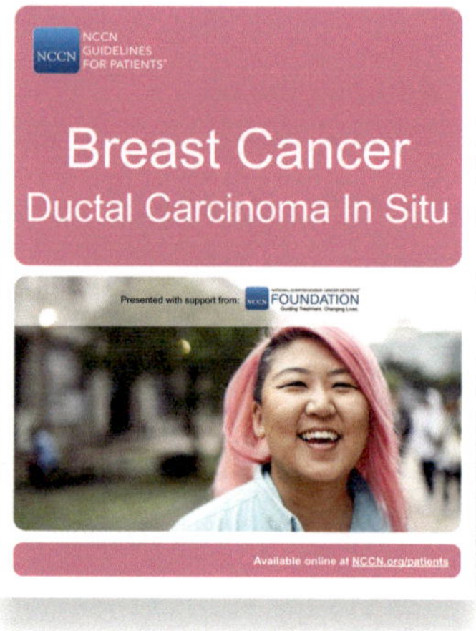

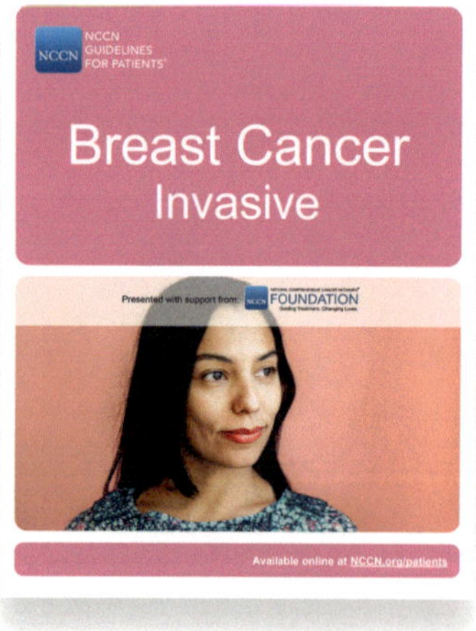

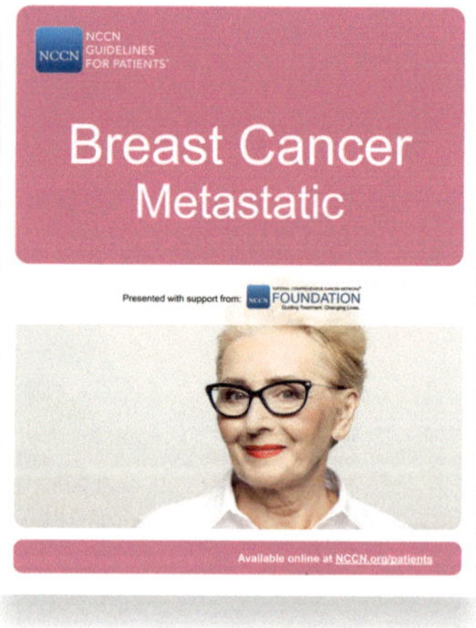

Early detection

Breast cancer screening aims to find breast cancer early. Breast cancer found earlier is treated more successfully, reducing the risk of dying from breast cancer. This book will cover screening recommendations for those assigned female at birth. It will also discuss screening and testing options for those who are pregnant or lactating (breastfeeding), and those with breast pain, nipple discharge, changes in the skin, lumps, or other symptoms that require further testing.

Transgender individuals

Due to lack of evidence, this book does not provide screening guidance for transgender individuals. Transgender individuals should consult with their primary care physician to determine when/whether screening would be appropriate.

Those assigned male at birth

Those assigned male at birth do not undergo regular mammogram screening. However, if you have breast pain or redness, or a change in the size and shape of one breast, then see your health care provider and read about recommended tests in Chapter 5.

Health care providers

During regular health checkups and breast cancer screening, you might come in contact with the following health care providers (HCPs):

- **Breast specialist** is an expert in breast health and disease.
- **Breast diagnostic radiologist** interprets the results of mammograms, MRIs, and other imaging tests, and performs needle biopsies as needed.
- **Gynecologist** diagnoses and treats diseases of the female reproductive organs.
- **Lactation consultant** specializes in breastfeeding.
- **Mammogram, MRI, and ultrasound technologists** operate the mammogram unit, or MRI or ultrasound machine.
- **Advanced practice providers** are nurse practitioners, physician assistants, and certified nurse midwives who can help prevent, evaluate, examine, and diagnose human disease, including breast cancer.
- **Obstetrician** specializes in pregnancy and in childbirth.
- **Pathologist** analyzes the cells, tissues, and organs removed during a biopsy or surgery.
- **Primary care provider (PCP)** or physician gives a wide range of care, including prevention and treatment.

Key points

- Anyone can develop breast cancer, but breast cancer occurs much more frequently in persons assigned female at birth.
- Inside breasts are lobules, ducts, fat, blood and lymph vessels, ligaments, and connective tissue. Lobules are structures that make breast milk. Ducts carry breast milk from the lobules to the nipple.
- Breast cancer often starts in the ducts or lobules and then spreads into the surrounding tissue.
- Breast cancer screening aims to find cancer early and before symptoms start. Breast cancer found earlier can be treated more successfully.

Breast cancer screening saves lives by detecting cancer earlier, when it can be treated more successfully.

"When I first discovered the small hard pebble under the skin of my chest wall, I felt sort of silly asking for so much testing for such a tiny bump. But, nearly 10 years later, I realize that this changed my life and may be the reason why I am still here today!"

2
Screening and diagnostic tests

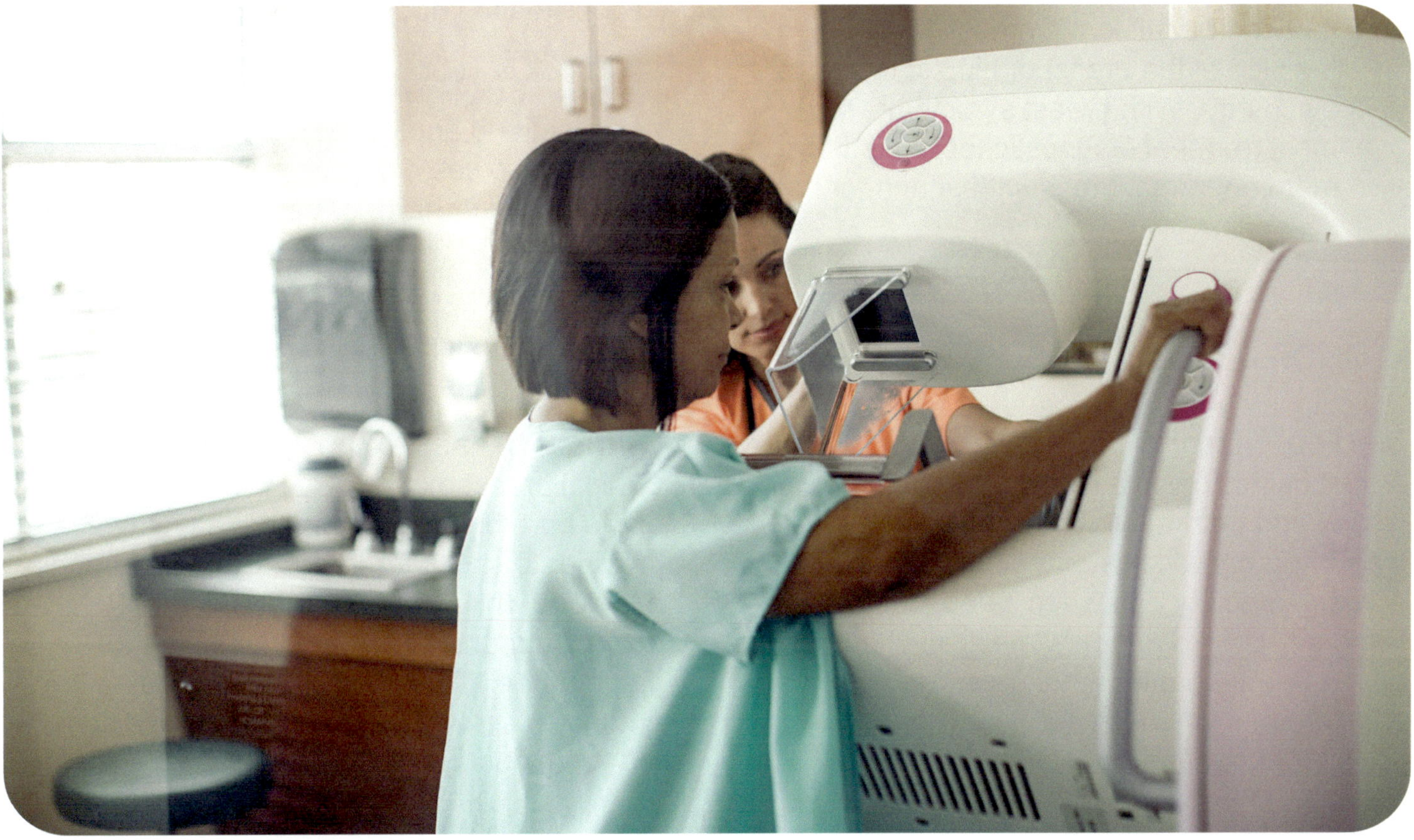

This chapter provides an overview of the various imaging tests used from breast cancer screening and diagnosis. Ask questions and keep copies of your test results. Online patient portals are a great way to access your test results.

What is the difference between screening and diagnostic tests?

- Screening is done on a regular basis when there are no symptoms. For example, an annual screening mammogram is done once a year to detect breast cancer before you have symptoms or anything abnormal before you have symptoms.
- Diagnostic tests are done when there are signs or symptoms such as a lump that can be felt in the breast, changes in the skin of the breast or nipple, or nipple discharge. With breast symptoms, the most frequent diagnostic tests used are mammograms, breast ultrasound, or both.

General health tests

Medical history

A medical history is a record of all health issues and treatments you have had in your life. Be prepared to list any illness, prior surgery, or injury and when it happened. Bring a list of old and new medicines and any over-the-counter medicines, herbals, or supplements you take. Tell your health care provider about any symptoms you have. A medical or health history will help determine which treatment is best for you.

Family history

Some cancers and other diseases can run in families. Your health care provider will ask about the health history of family members who are blood relatives. This information is called a family history. Ask family members about their health issues like heart disease, cancer and type of cancer, and diabetes, and at what age they were diagnosed.

Physical exam

During a physical exam, your health care provider may:

- Check your temperature, blood pressure, pulse, and breathing rate.
- Check your weight and height.
- Listen to your lungs and heart.
- Look in your eyes, ears, nose, and throat.
- Feel and apply pressure to parts of your body to see if organs are of normal size, are soft or hard, or cause pain when touched.
- Feel for enlarged lymph nodes in your neck, underarm, and groin.

Clinical breast exam

Clinical breast exam (CBE) is a physical exam of the bare breast performed by a health care provider to check for lumps or other changes. It is done while you are seated and/or lying down. Your provider should take time to palpate (feel) the entire breast, including the armpit. A nurse or assistant might also be in the room during the exam.

Family health information can change. Share with your provider any changes to your health or family history.

Mammogram

A mammogram is a picture of the inside of your breast. The picture is made using x-rays. A computer combines the x-rays to make detailed pictures.

Screening mammograms are annual preventive exams. Diagnostic mammograms are done when there are signs or symptoms in the breast or armpit. A diagnostic mammogram is more detailed than a screening mammogram. A screening mammogram only takes about 10 to 20 minutes, while a diagnostic mammogram can be longer.

Both screening and diagnostic mammograms use low-dose x-rays to examine the breast. They may use either the standard 2-dimensional (2D) digital mammography or 3-dimensional (3D) mammograms known as tomosynthesis.

A mammogram is performed on an outpatient basis. During mammography, a specially trained technologist will position your breast in the mammography unit. Your breast will be placed on a platform and compressed with a clear plastic paddle.

The breast is compressed in order to:

- Even out the breast thickness
- Spread out the tissue
- Hold the breast still
- Increase sharpness of the picture

You will be asked to stand very still and may need to hold your breath for a few seconds while the pictures are being taken. You will be asked to change positions between images. The process will be repeated for the other breast.

Screening mammogram

A screening mammogram is the only imaging test that has been found to reduce death from breast cancer. It is a test that uses low-dose x-rays to take four standard pictures of your breast (two on each side). A radiologist then reviews the images and determines if you need additional imaging. If you need additional imaging, you will likely have a diagnostic mammogram.

Diagnostic mammogram

A diagnostic mammogram might be done after a screening mammogram or for an abnormal finding such as a breast lump or nipple discharge. A radiologist will evaluate the diagnostic mammogram while you wait so if additional breast imaging is needed, it can be done right away. Diagnostic mammograms include extra compression in certain areas of the breast, magnification views, or rolling the breast to image additional areas of the breast.

Tomosynthesis

Tomosynthesis, or 3D mammograms, are a newer type of digital mammogram that may help to see small abnormal areas of the breast more easily. It takes multiple thin images that are then put together to make a complete picture. Tomosynthesis can decrease call back rates (the need for additional x-rays) and improve cancer detection. This is why 3D mammograms are recommended, if available in your area.

Contrast-enhanced mammogram

Contrast-enhanced mammography is a new technology that uses contrast material to improve the pictures of the inside of the breast. For those at increased risk for breast cancer, contrast-enhanced screening mammogram is an option.

Dense breasts

Breasts are composed of fat and soft tissue. Dense breasts have more soft tissue than fat. Having dense breast tissue may make it harder to see breast cancer or other changes in the breast on a mammogram. It can also increase your risk of developing breast cancer. If you have dense breast tissue, your HCP should discuss the risks and benefits of additional screening.

Your mammogram report will also include an assessment of your breast density, which is a description of how much fibrous and glandular tissue is in your breasts, as compared to fatty tissue. The denser your breasts, the harder it can be to see abnormal areas on mammograms. Having dense breasts also slightly raises your risk of getting breast cancer.

Mammogram findings

Calcifications

Calcifications are deposits of calcium in the tissues. Calcification in the breast can be seen on a mammogram, but cannot be detected by touch.

There are 2 types of breast calcification:

- **Macrocalcifications** are large deposits and are usually not related to cancer.
- **Microcalcifications** are specks of calcium that may be found in an area of rapidly dividing cells. Many microcalcifications clustered together may be a sign of cancer.

Distortion

This term describes when an area of the breast tissue appears at an odd angle, fuzzy or misshapened on a mammogram, particularly when compared to the other breast. This may just be due to how the breast was positioned during the mammogram. It might also be caused by a prior injury, procedure done on the breast, or a breast cancer.

Masses

A mass is an area of abnormal breast tissue. A mass could be solid, fluid-filled (cyst), or a combination of both. A mass might be seen with or without calcifications. Some masses can be watched over time with regular mammograms or ultrasound to see if they change, but others may need to be checked with a biopsy.

Asymmetries

Asymmetries are white areas seen on a mammogram that look different from the normal breast tissue pattern, particularly when compared to the other breast. Different types of asymmetries include focal asymmetry, developing asymmetry, and global asymmetry. Further imaging will likely be needed to get a better look at the area.

Ultrasound

An ultrasound (US) uses high-energy sound waves to form pictures of the inside of the body. This is similar to the sonogram used for pregnancy. Ultrasound does not use x-rays. It is frequently used without mammogram for diagnosis of breast symptoms in those under 30 years of age or with mammogram in those 30 years of age and over.

What's the difference between a screening and diagnostic mammogram?

A mammogram is a picture of the inside of your breast made using x-rays. During a mammogram, the breast is pressed between two plates while you stand in different positions. Multiple x-rays will be taken. A computer combines the x-rays to make detailed pictures.

- Screening mammograms are done on a regular basis when there are no signs or symptoms of breast cancer. Results take a few days.
- Diagnostic mammograms are used for those who have symptoms such as a lump, pain, nipple thickening or discharge, or whose breasts have changed shape or size.
- Diagnostic mammograms are also used to take a closer look at an abnormal area found in a screening mammogram.
- A radiologist will evaluate the diagnostic mammogram while you wait so if additional testing is needed, it can be done right away.
- Both types of mammograms use low-dose x-rays to examine the breast. They may use either the standard 2-dimensional (2D) digital mammography or 3-dimensional (3D) mammograms known as tomosynthesis.

Other imaging tests

Breast MRI

A magnetic resonance imaging (MRI) scan uses radio waves and powerful magnets to take pictures of the inside of the body. MRI does not use radiation. If needed, an MRI would be used in addition to a mammogram. If you are at high risk for breast cancer, an annual breast MRI might be recommended. Because of the very strong magnets used in the MRI machine, tell the technologist if you have any metal in your body.

Contrast material will be used to improve the pictures of the breast. For a breast MRI, a gadolinium-based contrast agent (GBCA)–a rare, heavy metal–is used to enhance the quality of the MRI. There are no harmful effects from GBCA, but it may linger in the body for months to years afterward. Talk to your doctor if you have any concerns.

Also, tell your care team if you have had allergic reactions to contrast in the past. This is important. You might be given medicines to avoid the effects of those allergies.

Breast sections

Quadrants are used to describe tumor location. Each breast is divided into 4 sections or quadrants. They are the upper outer quadrant (near the armpit), the upper inner quadrant (near the center of the body), the lower outer quadrant, and the lower inner quadrant. The nipple area is called the nipple-areola complex (NAC).

https://commons.wikimedia.org/wiki/File:Breast_quadrants.svg

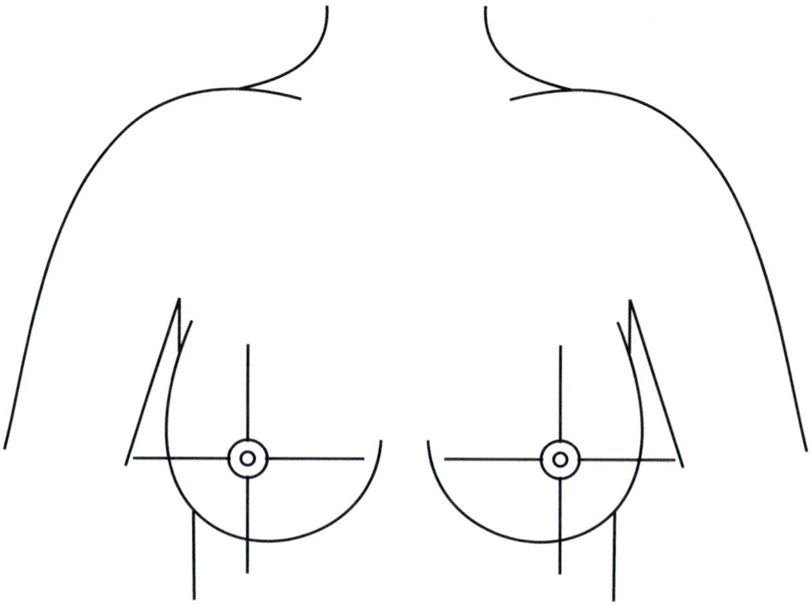

Tell your HCP about all of your medical conditions, including:

- If you are pregnant or think you might be pregnant
- The date of your last MRI with gadolinium
- If you have a gadolinium allergy or allergy to other x-ray contrast
- If you have any metal in your body (such as implanted infusion ports, metal screws or plates, some cardiac pacemakers, etc.)
- If you have kidney problems

Molecular breast imaging

Molecular breast imaging uses a radioactive tracer and special camera to find breast cancer. Molecular imaging such as breast-specific gamma imaging or sestamibi scan may improve detection. However, whole body radiation dose is much higher than that of standard mammograms. Molecular breast imaging is not a common breast screening imaging test.

What is your family cancer health history?

Some cancers and other diseases run in families – those who are related to you through genes passed down from parent to child. This information is called a family health history. Ask blood relatives about their health issues like heart disease, cancer, and diabetes, and at what age they were diagnosed. For relatives who were diagnosed with cancer, ask them (or other relatives if they are no longer living) what type of cancer they had, if they died from the cancer, and at what age the cancer was diagnosed.

Start by asking your parents, siblings, and children. Next, talk to half-siblings, aunts and uncles, nieces and nephews, grandparents, and grandchildren.

Write down what you learn about your family history and share with your health care provider.

Some of the questions to ask include:

- How old were you when each of these diseases and health conditions was diagnosed?
- What is our family's ancestry – from what countries did our ancestors originate?

BI-RADS

Mammographic density

Breast Imaging Reporting and Data System or BI-RADS is a standard system used to describe mammogram findings and results. A radiologist will categorize your mammogram results using a numbered system of 0 through 6. Talk to your health care provider about your mammogram results and what you need to do next.

These same BI-RADS categories can also be used to describe the results of a breast ultrasound or breast MRI.

BI-RADS also classifies breast density into groups, which are described next. See Guide 1.

BI-RADS 1

Negative

BI-RADS 1 means the test is negative for cancer. This is a normal test result. Your breasts look similar in the appearance of the breast tissue on the mammogram. There are no masses (lumps), distorted structures, or suspicious calcifications. In this case, negative means nothing new or abnormal was found.

BI-RADS 2

Benign (non-cancerous) finding

This is also a negative test result (there's no sign of cancer), but the radiologist chooses to describe a finding that is not cancer, such as benign calcifications, masses, or lymph nodes in the breast that are clearly not cancer. This can also be used to describe changes from a prior procedure (such as a biopsy) or surgery in the breast. This ensures that others who look at the mammogram in the future will not mistake the benign finding as suspicious.

Guide 1 BI-RADS findings
BI-RADS 1 is a negative (normal) result
BI-RADS 2 is a benign (non-cancerous) finding
BI-RADS 3 is a probable benign finding – follow-up in a short time frame is suggested
BI-RADS 4 is a suspicious abnormality – biopsy should be considered
BI-RADS 5 is highly suggestive of cancer – biopsy is strongly recommended
BI-RADS 6 is a biopsy-confirmed cancer

BI-RADS 3

Probably benign finding – Follow-up in a short time frame is suggested

A finding in this category has a very low (no more than 2%) chance of being cancer. It is not expected to change over time. But since it's not proven to be benign, breast experts agree that it is very safe to see if the area in question does change over time.

You will likely need follow-up with repeat imaging in 6 to 12 months and regularly after that until the finding is known to be stable (usually at least 2 years). This approach helps avoid unnecessary biopsies, but if the area does change over time, it still allows for early diagnosis.

BI-RADS 4

Suspicious abnormality – Biopsy should be considered

These findings do not definitely look like cancer but could be cancer. The radiologist is concerned enough to recommend a biopsy. The findings in this category can have a wide range of suspicion levels. For this reason, this category is often divided further:

- **4A:** Finding with a low likelihood of being cancer (more than 2% but no more than 10%)
- **4B:** Finding with a moderate likelihood of being cancer (more than 10% but no more than 50%)
- **4C:** Finding with a high likelihood of being cancer (more than 50% but less than 95%), but not as high as Category 5

BI-RADS 5

Highly suggestive of malignancy – Appropriate action should be taken

The findings look like cancer and have a high chance (at least 95%) of being cancer. Biopsy is very strongly recommended.

BI-RADS 6

Known biopsy-proven malignancy – Appropriate action should be taken

This category is used only for findings on a mammogram (or ultrasound or MRI) that have already been shown to be cancer by a previous biopsy. Imaging may be used in this way to see how well the cancer is responding to treatment.

We want your feedback!

Our goal is to provide helpful and easy-to-understand information on cancer.

Take our survey to let us know what we got right and what we could do better:

NCCN.org/patients/feedback

Key points

- Screening is done on a regular basis when there are no symptoms.
- Diagnostic tests are done when there are signs or symptoms.
- Clinical breast exam (CBE) is a physical exam of the bare breast performed by a health care provider to check for lumps or other changes.
- Both screening and diagnostic mammograms use low-dose x-rays to examine the breast. They may use either the standard 2-dimensional (2D) digital mammography or 3-dimensional (3D) mammograms known as tomosynthesis.
- Breast Imaging Reporting and Data System or BI-RADS is a standard system used to describe mammogram findings and results.
- These same BI-RADS categories can also be used to describe the results of a breast ultrasound or breast MRI.
- A magnetic resonance imaging (MRI) scan uses radio waves and powerful magnets to take pictures of the inside of the body.
- An ultrasound (US) uses high-energy sound waves to form pictures of the inside of the body.

"

My gynecologist never conducted a breast exam. I didn't even know it should be done! Fortunately, because of annual mammograms, my cancer was found early and I am now cancer-free."

3

Risk assessment for screening

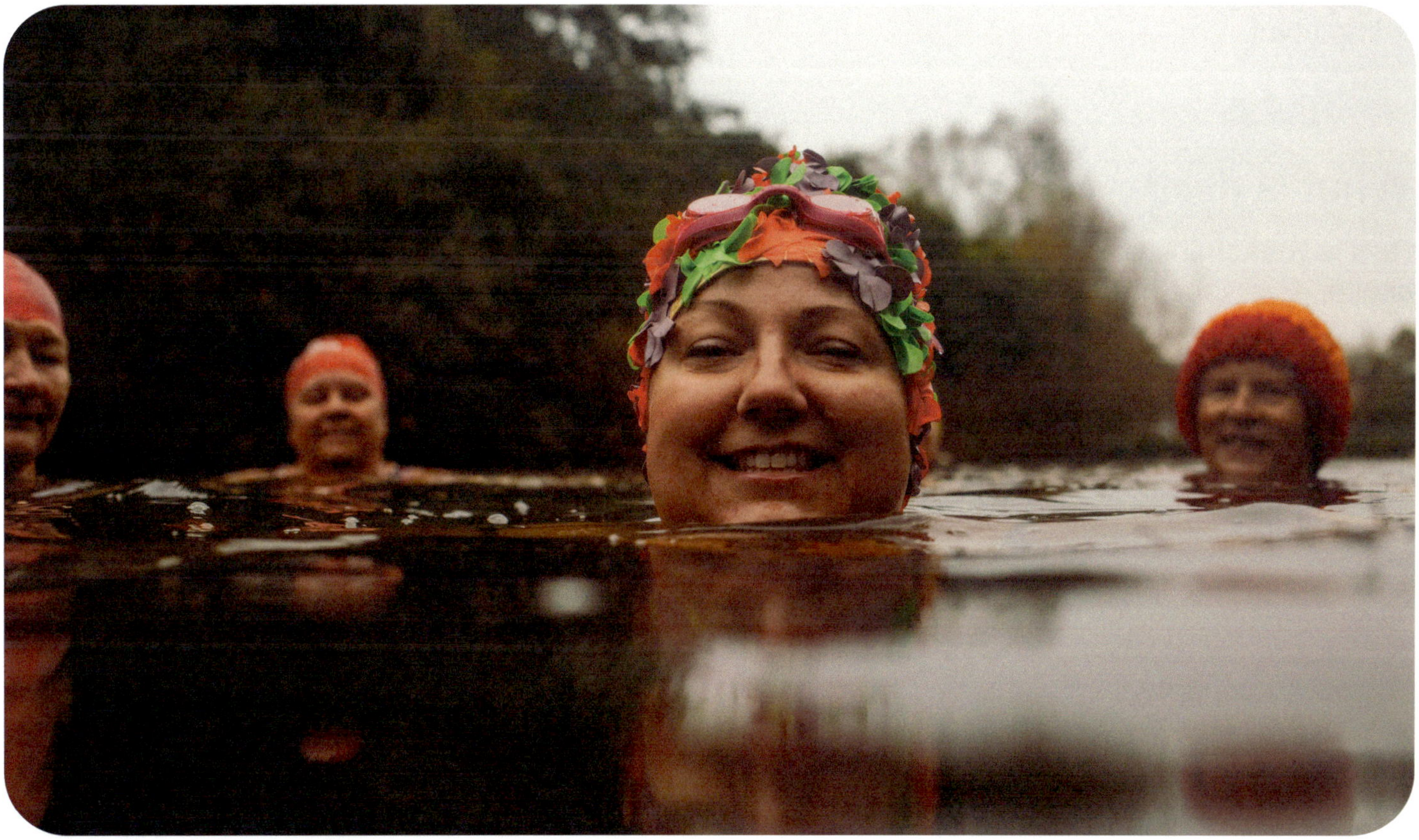

Risk is your chance for developing breast cancer. Everyone has some risk of developing breast cancer. However, some people are at increased risk for breast cancer and will have different screening recommendations. Screening mammograms are done for those assigned female at birth who do not have any signs or symptoms of breast cancer. More information on risk and screening recommendations can be found in this chapter.

See your health care provider (HCP) regularly for checkups. You might be asked to see your HCP more than every year based on your risk factors for developing breast cancer. Know your breasts and immediately report any changes to your HCP. As your family health history changes, keep your HCP updated. This is important.

What is risk?

Risk is your chance of developing breast cancer. Everyone has some risk for developing breast cancer. However, some people are at increased risk. Increased risk is based on your family history of certain cancers like ovarian and pancreatic cancer—not just breast cancer.

Other factors that put you at increased risk include:

- If you had radiation therapy (RT) to the chest between 10 and 30 years of age
- If you had a previous breast biopsy that showed atypical ductal hyperplasia (ADH) or a lobular neoplasia such as lobular carcinoma in situ (LCIS) or atypical lobular hyperplasia (ALH)
- Family history or genetic testing that suggests a genetic predisposition to breast, ovarian, or pancreatic cancer
- If you have a gene that predisposes you to breast cancer such a *BRCA1* or *BRCA2*

A risk assessment is based on your age, reproductive history (such as when your period started, if you have given birth and the age at which you first gave birth), and factors listed above. Individuals should undergo breast cancer risk assessment by 25 years of age. Your HCP should share information regarding potential benefits, risks, and limitations of breast screening. Shared decision-making between you and your HCP is encouraged.

There is no upper age limit for screening mammograms. This means that screening mammograms can continue throughout your entire life unless you and your provider decide otherwise based on your health.

Average risk

Average risk means you have no known genetic or family history that suggests you are at increased risk of developing breast cancer. It is recommended you have annual screening mammograms starting at 40 years of age. However, based on certain risk factors or as your family health history information changes, your HCP might recommend you start annual screening mammograms sooner. Annual means every year. If you have questions or concerns, ask your HCP.

25 to 39 years of age

See your HCP for a checkup every 1 to 3 years. This should include breast cancer risk assessment and, if not recently done, a breast exam.

40 years of age and over

See your HCP for a checkup every year. This should include ongoing breast cancer risk assessment and, if not recently done, a breast exam. Have an annual screening mammogram. If available, a tomosynthesis (3D mammogram) is recommended.

What is your risk level?

Cancer risk is largely based on a family history of cancer. The goal is to undergo a risk assessment by 25 years of age. This will determine when you should start annual screening mammograms. Your risk for developing breast cancer will be rated as average or increased risk.

Your level of risk is calculated based on the following information:

- What is your age?
- What is your race and ethnicity?
- What was the age of your first menstrual period (menarche)?
- Have you even been pregnant or given birth? What was your age when you first gave birth?
- How many biological relatives (parents, brothers, sisters, children, aunts, uncles, grandparents) on either side of your family have breast cancer? Are there other cancers such as ovarian, tubal, uterine, pancreatic, or prostate cancers in the family? What is/was the cancer stage or cancer cell type? At what age were they diagnosed?
- Have you had a breast biopsy? How many and when? Do you have a copy of the results?
- Have you or any close biological relatives had genetic testing? What were the results?
- Have you had a breast biopsy that showed atypical hyperplasia or lobular carcinoma in situ?

Increased risk

If you are at increased risk for developing breast cancer, see your HCP at least once a year. You might be asked to see your HCP more often.

Increased risk is for those who have or had:

- A strong family history that shows your lifetime risk is 20% or greater, when calculated using a risk assessment tool. Residual lifetime risk is based on the number of years of life that remain.
- Chest radiation therapy (RT) between 10 and 30 years of age
- 5-year risk of invasive breast cancer as calculated by the Gail model
- Atypical ductal hyperplasia (ADH), lobular carcinoma in situ (LCIS), or atypical lobular hyperplasia (ALH) and 20% or greater residual lifetime risk
- If you have a family history of breast cancer or family history that suggests genetic predisposition to breast, ovarian, or pancreatic cancer, or there is a known genetic mutation, then you will be referred to a genetic counselor or other health care professional who is an expert in cancer genetics. Consider submitting a saliva or blood specimen for genetic testing.

Increased risk

Residual lifetime risk of 20% or greater largely due to family history

Genetic predisposition

Known family history of breast cancer or family history that suggests genetic predisposition to breast, ovarian, or pancreatic cancer

Atypical ductal hyperplasia (ADH), lobular carcinoma in situ (LCIS), or atypical lobular hyperplasia (ALH) and 20% or greater residual lifetime risk

Previous radiation therapy

Chest radiation therapy (RT) between 10 and 30 years of age

5-year risk of invasive breast cancer as calculated by Gail model

If your residual lifetime risk is 20% or more

Individuals should undergo breast cancer risk assessment by 25 years of age. If your residual lifetime risk is 20 percent (20%) or more, then see your HCP for a checkup every 6 to 12 months. Ask your HCP about how you can reduce your risk of developing breast cancer.

Recommendations for screening will include an annual screening mammogram and/or breast MRI that will usually start before 40 years of age. When to start is based on family history and, typically, 7 to 10 years prior to when the youngest family member was diagnosed with breast cancer.

- Annual mammogram screening for those at increased risk might begin as early as 30 years of age.
- Annual breast MRI for those at increased risk might begin as early as 25 years of age. If breast MRI is not available or you cannot have an MRI, you can consider contrast-enhanced mammography or whole breast ultrasound.

You might be referred to a

- Genetic counselor or other health professional with expertise and experience in cancer genetics, if not already done
- Breast specialist

If you had chest RT between 10 and 30 years of age

If you had chest RT between 10 and 30 years of age, screening starts 8 years after radiation therapy (RT) ended. See your HCP for a checkup every year.

If you are currently 25 years of age or over, then

- See your HCP for a checkup every 6 to 12 months.
- Get an annual screening mammogram but not before 30 years of age. Tomosynthesis (3D mammogram) is recommended, if available.
- Consider an annual breast MRI but not before 25 years of age. A contrast-enhanced mammography or whole breast ultrasound might be an option for those who cannot undergo an MRI.
- Ask your HCP about how you can reduce your risk of developing breast cancer.

If you are at risk for invasive breast cancer based on the Gail model

Once you have been identified as being at high risk for developing invasive breast cancer, then

- See your HCP for a checkup every 6 to 12 months.
- Get an annual screening mammogram. Tomosynthesis (3D mammogram) is recommended, if available.
- Ask your HCP about how you can reduce your risk of developing breast cancer.

If you had ADH, LCIS, or ALH

If you had atypical ductal hyperplasia (ADH) or a lobular neoplasia such as lobular carcinoma in situ (LCIS) or atypical lobular hyperplasia (ALH), then

- See your HCP for a checkup every 6 to 12 months.
- Get an annual screening mammogram. Tomosynthesis (3D mammogram) is recommended, if available. Mammogram should start at the age you are diagnosed, but not before 30 years of age.
- Consider an annual breast MRI to begin when diagnosed but not before 25 years of age. A contrast-enhanced mammography or whole breast ultrasound might be an option for those who cannot undergo an MRI.
- Ask your HCP about how you can reduce your risk of developing breast cancer.

Key points

- Risk is your chance of developing breast cancer. Everyone has some risk for developing breast cancer.
- Screening mammograms are done for those born female who do not have any signs or symptoms of breast cancer.
- Annual screening mammograms are recommended to start at 40 years of age for those at average risk of developing breast cancer.
- For those at increased risk, annual screening mammograms may start as early as 30 years of age.
- For those at increased risk, annual breast MRIs may start as early as 25 years of age.
- Know your breasts and immediately report any changes to your health care provider (HCP).
- Ask your HCP about how you can reduce your risk of developing breast cancer.

Annual screening mammograms should start at 40 years of age for those at average risk.

4 Testing during pregnancy and breastfeeding

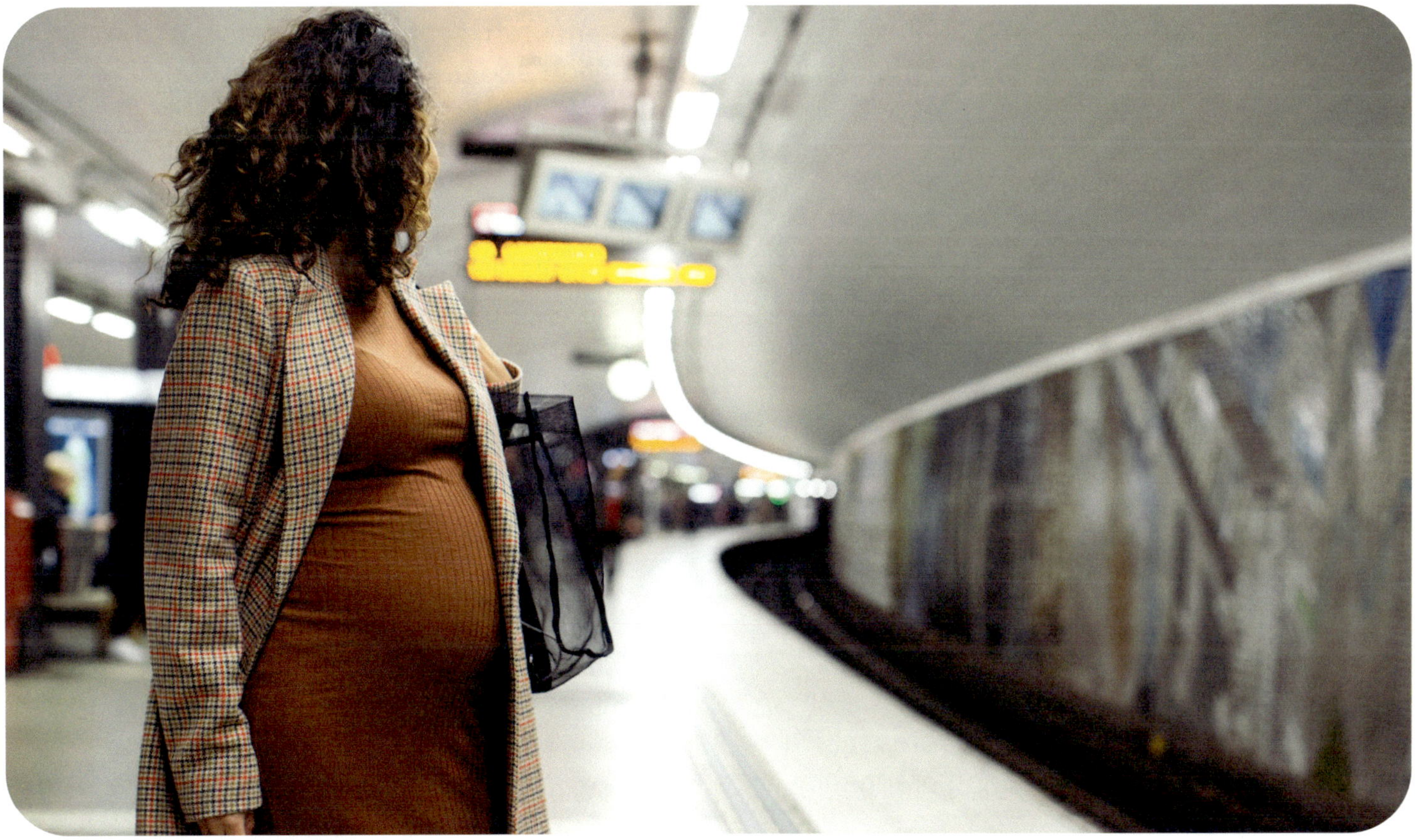

Pregnancy-associated breast cancer (PABC) is breast cancer that occurs during pregnancy, while breastfeeding, or within 1 year of delivery. It is important to continue taking care of your breast health during pregnancy and breastfeeding. Contact your health care provider about new or unusual changes to your breasts.

Overview

Changes in the breast are normal during pregnancy and breastfeeding (lactation). However, these changes can make it harder to detect small breast cancers. This is why it is important to continue taking care of your breast health. Delayed diagnosis of breast cancer during pregnancy or breastfeeding does happen. This may result in more advanced disease, larger tumors, and a greater likelihood of cancer in the lymph nodes.

Pregnancy-associated breast cancer (PABC) is defined as breast cancer occurring during pregnancy, while breastfeeding, or within one year of delivery. While rare, PABC is the most common invasive cancer diagnosed during pregnancy.

See your health care provider (HCP) regularly for checkups. Contact your HCP for any new or worsening changes.

Breast cancer screening during pregnancy and lactation is similar to non-pregnant and non-lactating women with some exceptions. For example, due to safety concerns, breast MRI is not generally performed during pregnancy, although it can be safely used in lactating women. Breast ultrasound and mammography (with abdominal shielding) can be safely performed during pregnancy. So, breast screening, breast lumps, and other breast problems are evaluated with mammogram and ultrasound in a similar way during pregnancy and breastfeeding as they are in non-pregnant patients.

This section discusses screening recommendations during pregnancy and breastfeeding. It also provides information on signs and symptoms that you should report to your HCP.

During pregnancy

Clinical breast exams and breast cancer screening mammograms can and should continue on a yearly basis during pregnancy. Mammograms contain a very low level of radiation and are considered safe during pregnancy. Abdominal shielding should be used to reduce radiation exposure to the fetus.

Normal changes happen in the breast, skin, and nipple during pregnancy. However, if you notice anything new or unusual contact your HCP. For changes in the skin or breast such as persistent or focused pain, a lump, or nipple discharge an ultrasound will be done.

During breastfeeding

Clinical breast cancer exams and screening mammograms can and should continue on a yearly basis during breastfeeding (lactation). If you are at increased risk for developing breast cancer, then a breast MRI may be done.

Nursing or breast pumping before a mammogram is recommended.

Normal changes happen in the breast, skin, and nipple during lactation or breastfeeding. Contact your doctor if you notice any new or unusual changes to your breast or armpit, or if

- Your breast is warm to the touch, painful, or red in color.
- Your breast skin appears thickened with large pores (peau d'orange).
- You have breast pain.

Nipple changes

For changes in the nipple, contact your HCP if:

- Your nipple is retracted or pulled in (inverted) when it was not that way before.
- Your nipple has changed in shape.
- Your nipple becomes tender and it is not related to your menstrual cycle.
- Your nipple has skin changes.
- You have new nipple discharge.

It is important to keep follow-up visits and imaging test appointments. Seek good routine medical care, including preventive care and cancer screenings.

Key points

- An annual clinical breast exam (CBE) and mammogram are recommended during pregnancy and breastfeeding.
- Mammograms contain a very low level of radiation and are considered safe during pregnancy. Abdominal shielding should be used to reduce radiation exposure to the fetus.
- Nursing or breast pumping before a mammogram is recommended.
- Breast MRI is not recommended during pregnancy, but might be done in some cases during breastfeeding.
- Normal changes happen in the breast, skin, and nipple during lactation or breastfeeding. However, if you notice anything new or unusual contact your health care provider

5

What to do when there are symptoms

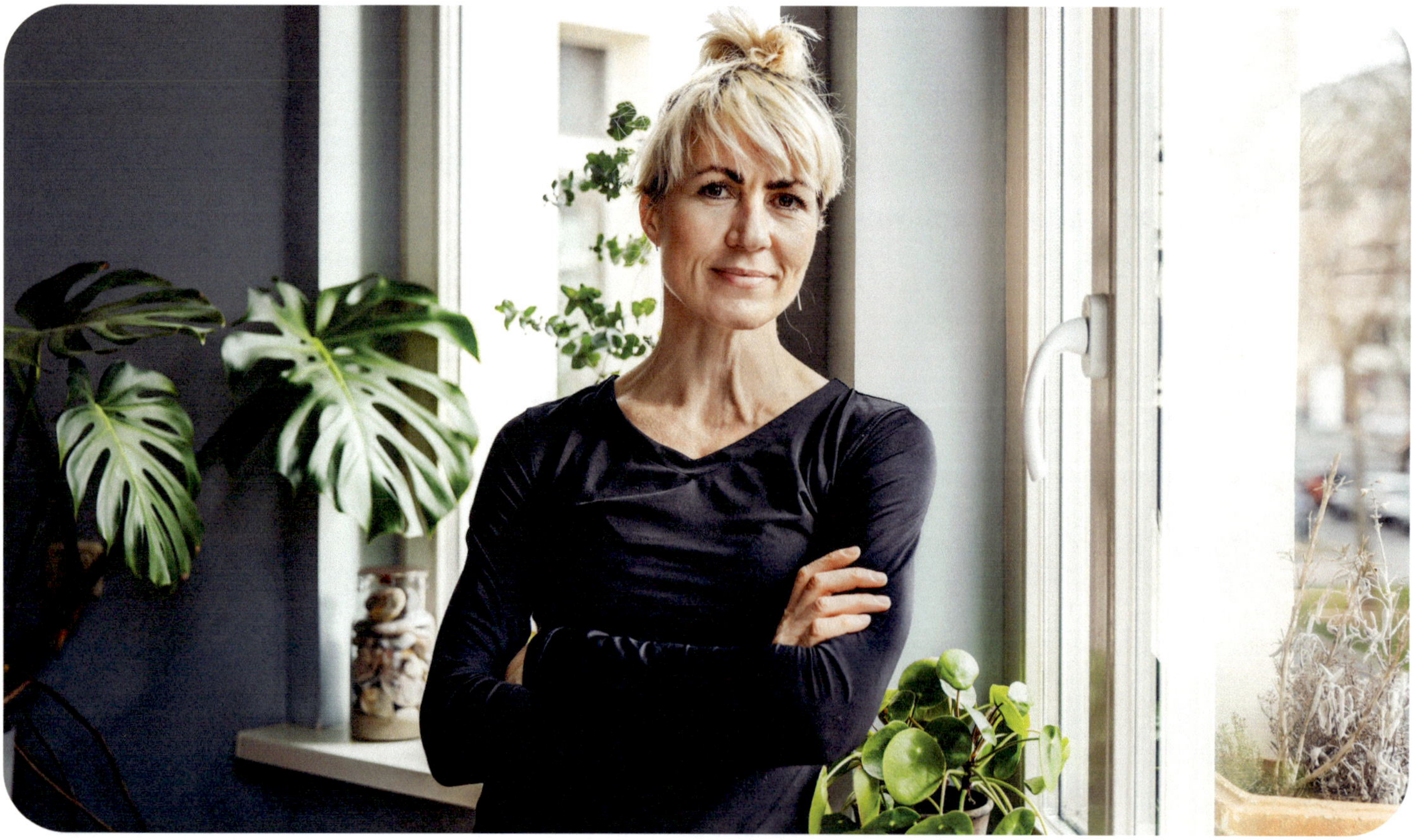

This chapter is for those with signs or symptoms that suggest further testing. Certain conditions are difficult to diagnose. See a breast specialist for any unusual symptoms or skin or nipple changes.

Signs and symptoms

A sign can be seen by someone else like your health care provider (HCP). A symptom is something only you can feel. If you have any signs or symptoms that might suggest breast cancer, another cancer or disease, you may have more tests. These are called diagnostic tests because they help diagnose a disease or condition. It is important to tell your HCP if something doesn't feel or look right and has been that way for a few days. Don't wait to say something!

Signs and symptoms that suggest further testing:

- Breast pain
- Lump, mass, nodules, or skin thickening that can be felt in the breast
- Enlarged breasts or gynecomastia (in those assigned male at birth)
- Lump or swelling in or near the armpit (axilla)
- Breast implant-related symptoms

Breast pain

Breast pain may be monitored to see if it persists, it is severe, and if there are changes in skin, or other symptoms such as a lump or nipple discharge. For pain that is focused or concentrated in one area, you may have an ultrasound. A mammogram might also be done if you are 30 years of age or over and you have not had a recent mammogram. Depending on the test results, further testing might be needed.

Lumps and other signs

If you have a symptom that can be felt (palpable) such as a lump, mass, nodules, or skin thickening, then

- For those under 30 years of age, an ultrasound is preferred as a diagnostic test. However, your doctor may wait and observe any changes for 1 to 2 menstrual cycles before ordering an ultrasound.
- For those 30 years of age or over, a diagnostic mammogram and ultrasound are recommended.

For a benign finding, you may not need any further evaluation. If the mammogram or ultrasound show something, your HCP may recommend a core needle biopsy, additional physical exams, or more frequent mammograms and/or ultrasounds to monitor the symptom. You are also an important part of monitoring and should let your HCP know if you notice any new changes. If you have any questions or concerns, talk with your HCP.

Lump in or near armpit

A diagnostic mammogram and ultrasound will be done for a lump or mass in or near the armpit (axilla). If you are under 30 years of age, a mammogram might only be done if the ultrasound results are unclear or cancer is suspected. Depending on your symptoms, you might be referred to a breast specialist.

Breast implant-related symptoms

Those with breast implants have a very small risk of developing breast implant-associated anaplastic large cell lymphoma (BIA-ALCL), a type of cancer. It is mostly seen in textured implants about 7 to 9 years after implantation. The main symptoms of BIA-ALCL are persistent swelling, or a lump or pain in the area of the breast implant. Since BIA-ALCL is so rare, only those with symptoms will undergo further testing.

If it has been more than 1 year since breast implant surgery and you are having symptoms related to the implants, then your health care provider should consult with a multidisciplinary team with experience in implant-related problems. If BIA-ALCL is suspected, then you will undergo further testing.

Skin changes

Skin changes include puckering, dimpling, a rash, or redness of the skin of the breast. Some people have a rash or redness of the nipple and the surrounding skin. The skin might look like an orange peel or the texture might feel different.

Some skin changes might be a sign of inflammatory breast cancer (IBC) or Paget disease. Since these diseases are difficult to diagnose, you might be referred to a breast specialist.

Know your breasts and immediately report any changes to your health care provider.

Possible inflammatory breast cancer

Inflammatory breast cancer (IBC) is a rare, aggressive cancer where cancer cells block lymph vessels in the skin of the breast. This causes the breast to look red and swollen and feel warm to the touch.

Possible signs of IBC:

- Peau d'orange (pitted or dimpled appearance of skin)
- Skin thickening (skin has an orange-peel texture)
- Edema (swelling caused by excess fluid in body tissue)
- Erythema (reddening of the skin, usually in patches)

If IBC is suspected, then a diagnostic mammogram will be done. An ultrasound might be done, too.

- For BI-RADS 1, 2, or 3, you might be referred to a breast specialist and/or have a breast MRI. A core needle biopsy or biopsy of the skin or nipple might be done.
- For BI-RADS 4 or 5, a core needle biopsy guided by imaging of the breast will be done.

More information on inflammatory breast cancer can be found in the *NCCN Guidelines for Patients: Breast Cancer – Invasive*, available at NCCN.org/patientguidelines.

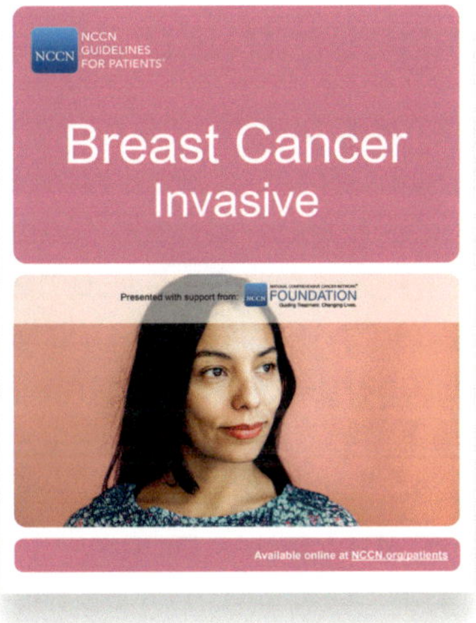

Possible Paget disease

In Paget disease, abnormal cells are found in the nipple. This can cause scaly rash, ulcers, bleeding, or itching of the nipple or areola.

Possible signs of Paget disease or other types of breast cancer:

- Nipple irritation or bleeding
- Scaly rash
- Skin ulcers

If Paget disease is suspected, then a diagnostic mammogram will be done. An ultrasound might be done, too.

- For BI-RADS 1, 2, or 3, you might be referred to a breast specialist and/or have a breast MRI. A core needle biopsy or biopsy of the skin or nipple might be done.
- For BI-RADS 4 or 5, a core needle biopsy guided by imaging of the breast will be done.

"Find a breast specialist if you have possible signs of inflammatory breast cancer (IBC)."

Nipple discharge

When fluid that is not milk comes from the nipple, it is called nipple discharge. Nipple discharge is common, and, in most cases unrelated to breast cancer.

For example, discharge can occur

- During pregnancy following breast stimulation
- In those with certain thyroid conditions, and
- In those taking certain medicines, such as estrogen, oral contraceptives, opiates, and certain blood pressure medicine
- Due to inflammatory conditions of the breast duct that is not related to cancer

Nipple discharge is normal during breastfeeding (lactation). Some women can express small amounts of yellow, green, or milky discharge if they squeeze the nipples. This is call expressed discharge. However, it is abnormal when the nipple discharge is any of the following:

- Spontaneous – occurs without squeezing or dried discharge is seen on your bra or other clothing
- Bloody or clear
- From a single duct opening on the nipple on only one breast

If you have abnormal nipple discharge without other symptoms, then

- For those under 30 years of age, an ultrasound will be done. A diagnostic mammogram might also be done.
- For those 30 years of age or over, a diagnostic mammogram and ultrasound will be done.

Depending on the BI-RADS result, you might have a core need biopsy, additional physical exams, more frequent mammograms and/or ultrasounds to monitor the symptom. You might be referred to a breast specialist and a breast MRI might be done. If you have any questions or concerns, talk with your health care provider (HCP).

Milky

For bilateral milky discharge, you might have an endocrine (hormone) workup. Milky discharge is generally normal in pregnancy.

Those assigned male at birth

Those assigned male at birth do not undergo routine screening mammograms. However, males can develop breast cancer. A diagnostic mammogram may be ordered if you have extra breast tissue (gynecomastia). If you have bloody nipple discharge or symptoms that can be felt such as a lump, then an ultrasound will be done in addition to the diagnostic mammogram. A core needle biopsy might also be done. Your condition will be monitored and you might be asked to return to your HCP for regular testing. Consider seeing a breast specialist.

Gynecomastia

Gynecomastia is the abnormal growth of breast tissue in those assigned male at birth. There might be concern if one breast appears enlarged. This is called asymmetrical gynecomastia. A diagnostic mammogram with possible ultrasound will be done.

Biopsy

A biopsy is a procedure that removes a sample of tissue. The sample is sent to a lab for testing. A pathologist will examine the biopsy under the microscope to determine if the tissue is benign (not cancer) or due to pre-cancer or cancer. Biopsy results can be found in a pathology report. Ask questions about your biopsy results and what it means for next steps.

Depending on the biopsy results, you may not need any additional testing and be returned to routine follow-up care. However, the biopsy results may require additional testing or more frequent exams or imaging. If cancer is found, you will be referred for cancer treatment.

There are different types of biopsies. Some biopsies are guided using imaging, such as a mammogram, ultrasound, or MRI. The primary or main area of concern is biopsied first. Other areas may also be biopsied.

Types of possible biopsies include:

- **Aspiration or core biopsy (CB)** uses needles of different sizes guided by imaging to remove a sample of tissue.
- **Excisional** removes a small amount of tissue through a cut in the skin or body (surgery).

Before biopsies are performed, usually the area is injected with numbing medicine. A core needle biopsy (CNB) removes more than one tissue sample, but usually through the same area on the breast. The samples are small. The needle is often guided into the tumor with imaging. When mammography is used during a biopsy, it is called a stereotactic needle biopsy.

Biopsy

In a biopsy, a sample of tumor is removed. There are different types of biopsy. This image shows an ultrasound-guided needle biopsy.

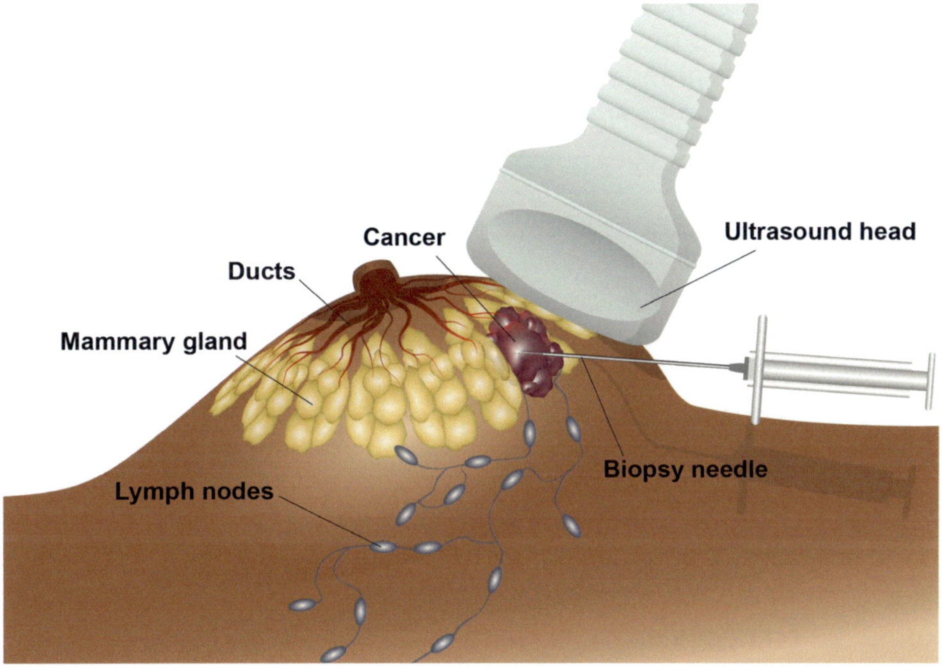

One or more clips may be placed near the breast tumor during a biopsy. The clips are small, painless, and made of metal. They will mark the site for future treatment and imaging. The clips stay in place until surgery. If the area biopsied is benign, the clip will remain in place to mark the biopsy site on future imaging. The clip causes no problems, even if they are left in place for a long time. You will be able to go through airport security.

There are both physical and emotional experiences in having biopsies. You may need to rest and place an ice pack on the biopsy area after the procedure. If you are working or have other commitments, you may want to take the day off to recover emotionally and physically from the experience.

Biopsy results

Histology is the study of the anatomy (structure) of cells, tissues, and organs under a microscope. It is used to make treatment decisions. Your pathology report will contain information about histology.

You may be recommended to have an open biopsy (surgery) to remove (excise) the tumor to confirm histology if core needle biopsy shows the following:

- Indeterminate
- Benign and image discordant (what is seen on the mammogram or ultrasound is not explained by what is seen under the microscope)
- Possible atypical ductal hyperplasia

Talk to your health care provider for more information on next steps.

Key points

- A sign can be seen by someone else like your health care provider. A symptom is something only you can feel like pain. If you have any signs or symptoms that might suggest breast cancer, another cancer or disease, you will have more tests.
- Some skin changes might be a sign of inflammatory breast cancer (IBC) or Paget disease. Because these diseases are difficult to diagnose you might be referred to a breast specialist.
- If IBC is suspected, then a diagnostic mammogram and possibly an ultrasound will be done. An MRI might be done, too.
- If Paget disease is suspected, then a diagnostic mammogram and possibly an ultrasound will be done. A skin punch biopsy may be done to remove a small sample of skin.
- Nipple discharge is common, and, in many cases unrelated to breast cancer.
- Those assigned male at birth do not undergo routine screening mammograms. However, a diagnostic mammogram will be done if you have extra breast tissue (gynecomastia). If you have bloody nipple discharge or symptoms that can be felt such as a lump, then an ultrasound will be done in addition to a diagnostic mammogram.
- A biopsy is a procedure that removes a sample of tissue for testing.
- Histology is the study of the anatomy (structure) of cells, tissues, and organs under a microscope.

6
Questions to ask

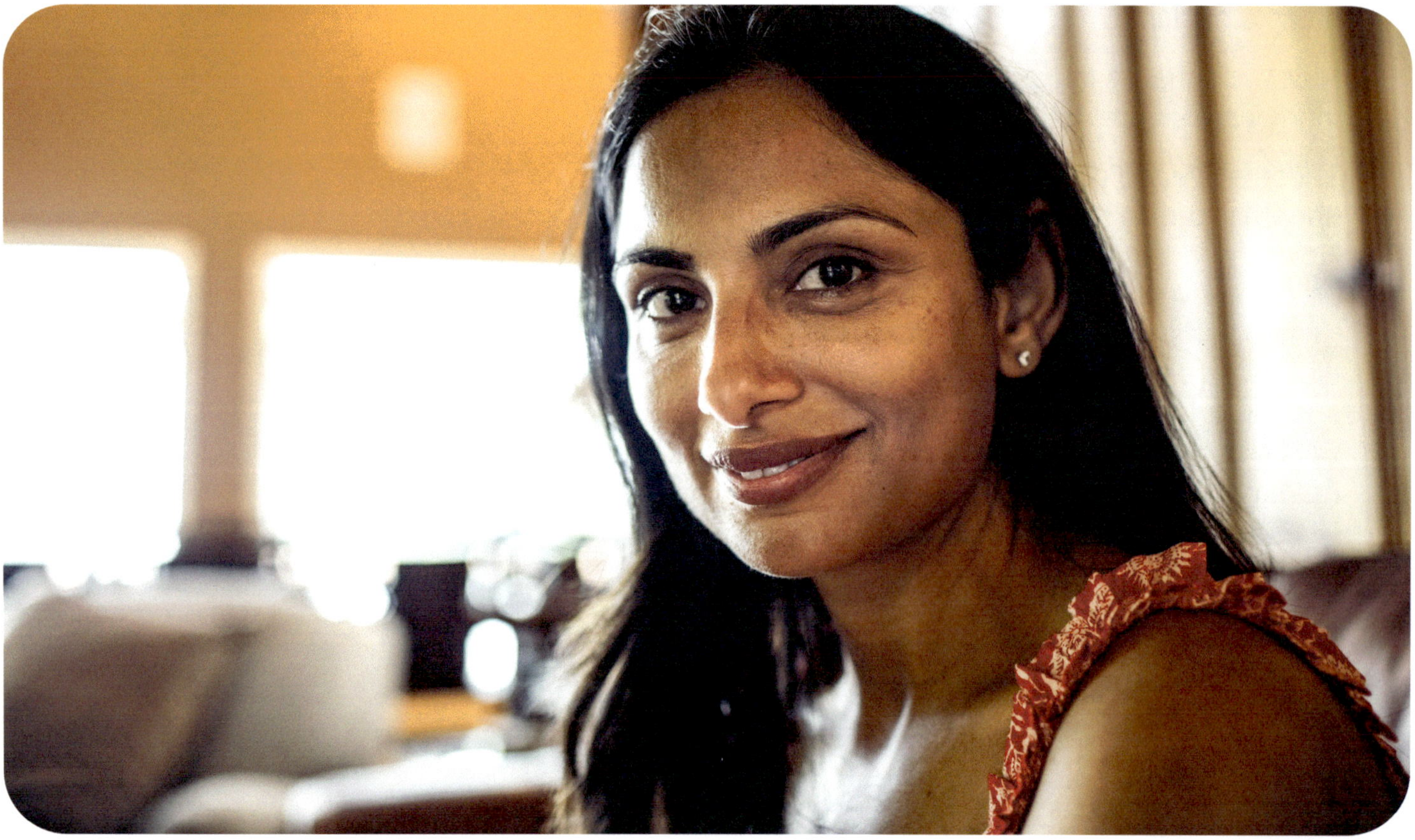

Questions to ask

In shared decision-making, you and your health care provider (HCP) discuss your risk for developing breast cancer and agree to a screening schedule. This chapter offers possible questions to ask your HCP and additional resources.

Questions to ask about risk

1. What is my risk for developing breast cancer? Am I at average or increased risk?
2. What can I do to lower my chances of developing breast cancer?
3. Based on my risk level, when should I start yearly screening mammograms?
4. If I am at increased risk, will I have both a screening mammogram and a breast MRI every year?
5. I don't know my family health history. How will this affect my risk assessment?
6. Breast cancer doesn't run in my family, but some family members have had cancer. Why might I be at increased risk for developing breast cancer?

Questions to ask about screening mammograms

1. Who will schedule my screening mammogram?
2. Will someone send me a reminder to schedule a mammogram?
3. Do I have a choice which type of screening mammogram to get?
4. How do I know what type of screening mammogram is being used?
5. Is there a fee or copay for screening mammograms? What about tomosynthesis (3D) screening mammograms?
6. Mammograms are stressful and uncomfortable. How can I prepare for this and worry less while waiting for the result?
7. I don't see the BI-RADS listed on my mammogram results. Where can I get that information?
8. How common are cysts? If cysts are benign, why does it seem concerning?
9. How will you make me comfortable during the mammogram if I am pregnant or breastfeeding?
10. Should I nurse or pump before the mammogram?

Questions to ask about testing and diagnosis

1. What tests will I have and why? How often will they be repeated? Will my insurance pay for these tests?
2. How should I prepare for testing?
3. What will you do to make me comfortable during testing?
4. What if I am pregnant or want to become pregnant? If I am breastfeeding?
5. When will I have a biopsy? Will I have more than one? What are the risks?
6. How will my biopsy be performed? What else might be done at this time?
7. How soon will I know the results and who will explain them to me?
8. How can I get a copy of the pathology report and other test results?
9. Who will talk with me about the next steps? When?
10. What can I do before my next appointment?

Resources

American Association for Cancer Research (AACR)
aacr.org

American Breast Cancer Foundation
youandbreastcancer.com/en-bc/home

American Cancer Society (ACS)
cancer.org/cancer/breast-cancer.html

cancer.org/cancer-information-in-other-languages/spanish.html

American Society of Clinical Oncology (ASCO)
cancer.net

Breast Cancer Alliance (BCA)
breastcanceralliance.org

Breast Cancer Portrait Project
breastcancerportraitproject.org

Breastcancer.org
breastcancer.org

Brem Foundation
bremfoundation.org

Cancer*Care*
cancercare.org

cancercare.org/espanol

Cancer Support Community
cancersupportcommunity.org/living-cancer

DiepCFoundation
diepcfoundation.org

FORCE - Facing Our Risk of Cancer Empowered
facingourrisk.org

GPAC - Global Patient Advocacy Coalition
GPACunited.org

HealthWell Foundation
healthwellfoundation.org

Inflammatory Breast Cancer Research Foundation
ibcresearch.org

MedlinePlus
medlineplus.gov

medlineplus.gov/spanish/

National Cancer Institute (NCI)
cancer.gov/types/breast

National Coalition for Cancer Survivorship
canceradvocacy.org/toolbox

National Financial Resource Directory
- Patient Advocate Foundation
patientadvocate.org/explore-our-resources/national-financial-resource-directory/

OncoLink
oncolink.org

Patient Access Network Foundation
panfoundation.org

Radiological Society of North America
radiologyinfo.org

SHARE Cancer Support
sharecancersupport.org

Sharsheret
sharsheret.org

Smart Patients
smartpatients.com/communities/breast-cancer

Susan G. Komen
komen.org

Testing.com
testing.com

The Male Breast Cancer Coalition
malebreastcancerhappens.org

Unite for HER
uniteforher.org

Young Survival Coalition (YSC)
youngsurvival.org

Let us know what you think!

Please take a moment to complete an online survey about the NCCN Guidelines for Patients.

NCCN.org/patients/response

Words to know

areola
A darker, round area of skin on the breast around the nipple.

atypical ductal hyperplasia (ADH)
A benign (not cancer) condition in which there are more cells than normal in the lining of breast ducts and the cells look abnormal under a microscope. Having atypical ductal hyperplasia increases the risk of breast cancer.

atypical lobular hyperplasia (ALH)
A benign condition in which there are more cells than normal in the breast lobules and the cells look abnormal under a microscope. Having atypical lobular hyperplasia increases the risk of breast cancer.

axillary lymph node (ALN)
A small disease-fighting structure that is near the armpit.

biopsy
A procedure that removes fluid or tissue samples to be tested for a disease.

calcification
Deposits of calcium in the tissues.

clinical breast exam (CBE)
A physical exam of the breast performed by a health care provider to check for lumps or other changes.

contrast
A substance put into your body to make clearer pictures during imaging tests.

core needle biopsy (CNB)
A procedure that removes tissue samples with a hollow needle. Also called core biopsy (CB).

diagnostic mammogram
Pictures of the insides of both breasts that are made from a set of x-rays in individuals with signs or symptoms.

duct
A tube-shaped structure through which milk travels to the nipple.

ductal carcinoma
A cancer derived from cells that line small tube-shaped vessels.

ductal carcinoma in situ (DCIS)
A breast cancer that has not grown outside the breast ducts.

edema
Swelling caused by excess fluid in body tissues.

erythema
Reddening of the skin, usually in patches.

excoriation
Skin that has worn off.

gene
Coded instructions in cells for making new cells and controlling how cells behave.

genetic counseling
Expert guidance on the chance for a disease that is passed down in families.

gynecomastia
The abnormal growth of breast tissue in those assigned male at birth.

hereditary breast cancer
Breast cancer that was likely caused by abnormal genes passed down from biological parent to child.

histology
The structure of cells, tissue, and organs as viewed under a microscope.

lobule
A gland in the breast that makes breast milk.

lobular carcinoma
A breast cancer that started in cells that line the milk glands (lobules).

lobular carcinoma in situ (LCIS)
A benign (not cancer) condition in which abnormal cells are found in the lobules of the breast.

lobular neoplasia
A benign condition in which abnormal cells are found in the lobules of the breast and increases the risk of developing breast cancer in the future. Types of lobular neoplasia include atypical lobular hyperplasia (ALH) and lobular carcinoma in situ (LCIS).

lymph
A clear fluid containing white blood cells.

lymph node
A small, bean-shaped disease-fighting structure.

lymphadenopathy
Lymph nodes that are abnormal in size or consistency.

lymphedema
Swelling in the body due to a buildup of fluid called lymph.

magnetic resonance imaging (MRI)
A test that uses radio waves and powerful magnets to make pictures of the inside of the body.

mammogram
A picture of the inside of the breast that is made by an x-ray test.

menopause
The point in time when menstrual periods end, typically diagnosed after 12 months of no periods.

nipple-areola complex (NAC)
The ring of darker breast skin is called the areola. The raised tip within the areola is called the nipple.

nipple discharge
Fluid that is not milk coming from the nipple.

palpable adenopathy
Lymph nodes that feel abnormal in size or consistency.

pathologist
An expert who interprets cells and tissues removed during a biopsy or surgery.

postmenopausal
The state of having no more menstrual periods.

premenopause
The state of having menstrual periods.

radiation therapy (RT)
A treatment that uses high-energy rays.

radiologist
Expert who interprets the results of mammograms, MRIs, and other imaging tests.

residual lifetime risk
Risk based on the number of years of life that remain.

screening mammogram
X-rays of the breasts taken to check for breast cancer in someone without signs or symptoms of cancer.

technologist
Person trained to operate a mammography unit to produce images of the breasts for diagnostic purposes.

ultrasound (US)
A test that uses sound waves to take pictures of the inside of the body.

Notes

NCCN Contributors

This patient guide is based on the NCCN Clinical Practice Guidelines in Oncology (NCCN Guidelines®) for Breast Cancer Screening and Diagnosis, Version 1.2022. It was adapted, reviewed, and published with help from the following people:

Dorothy A. Shead, MS
Senior Director
Patient Information Operations

Tanya Fischer, MEd, MSLIS
Senior Medical Writer

Susan Kidney
Senior Graphic Design Specialist

The NCCN Clinical Practice Guidelines in Oncology (NCCN Guidelines®) for Breast Cancer Screening and Diagnosis, Version 1.2022 were developed by the following NCCN Panel Members:

*Therese B. Bevers, MD/Chair
The University of Texas
MD Anderson Cancer Center

Mark Helvie, MD/Vice-Chair
University of Michigan
Rogel Cancer Center

Jennifer L. Baker, MD
UCLA Jonsson
Comprehensive Cancer Center

Debbie L. Bennett, MD
Siteman Cancer Center at Barnes-Jewish Hospital and Washington University School of Medicine

Ermelinda Bonaccio, MD
Roswell Park Comprehensive Cancer Center

Melissa S. Camp, MD
The Sidney Kimmel Comprehensive Cancer Center at Johns Hopkins

*Sona Chikarmane, MD
Dana-Farber/Brigham and Women's Cancer Center

Emily F. Conant, MD
Abramson Cancer Center
at the University of Pennsylvania

Mohammad Eghtedari, MD, PhD
UC San Diego Moores Cancer Center

William B. Farrar, MD
The Ohio State University Comprehensive Cancer Center - James Cancer Hospital and Solove Research Institute

Meghan R. Flanagan, MD, MPH
Fred Hutchinson Cancer Research Center/ Seattle Cancer Care Alliance

Randall E. Harris, MD, PhD
The Ohio State University Comprehensive Cancer Center - James Cancer Hospital and Solove Research Institute

Linda Hodgkiss, MD
St. Jude Children's Research Hospital/ The University of Tennessee Health Science Center

Tamarya L. Hoyt, MD
Vanderbilt-Ingram Cancer Center

Maxine S. Jochelson, MD
Memorial Sloan Kettering Cancer Center

Seema Khan, MD
Robert H. Lurie Comprehensive Cancer Center of Northwestern University

Rachael B. Lancaster, MD
O'Neal Comprehensive
Cancer Center at UAB

Constance D. Lehman, MD, PhD
Massachusetts General Hospital
Cancer Center

Jessica Maxwell, MD, MS
Fred & Pamela Buffett Cancer Center

Diana L. Miglioretti, PhD
UC Davis Comprehensive Cancer Center

Bethany L. Niell, MD, PhD
Moffitt Cancer Center

Bhavika K. Patel, MD
Mayo Clinic Cancer Center

*Mark Pearlman, MD
University of Michigan Rogel Cancer Center

Liane Philpotts, MD
Yale Cancer Center/Smilow Cancer Hospital

Donna Plecha, MD
Case Comprehensive Cancer Center/ University Hospitals Seidman Cancer Center and Cleveland Clinic Taussig Cancer Institute

Jennifer K. Plichta, MD, MS
Duke Cancer Institute

Mary Lou Smith, JD, MBA
Research Advocacy Network

Roberta M. Strigel, MD, MS
University of Wisconsin
Carbone Cancer Center

Lusine Tumyan, MD
City of Hope National Medical Center

Nicole S. Winkler, MD
Huntsman Cancer Institute
at the University of Utah

Dulcy E. Wolverton, MD
University of Colorado Cancer Center

NCCN Staff

Lisa Hang, PhD

Rashmi Kumar, PhD

Mary Anne Bergman

* Reviewed this patient guide. For disclosures, visit NCCN.org/disclosures.

NCCN Cancer Centers

Abramson Cancer Center
at the University of Pennsylvania
Philadelphia, Pennsylvania
800.789.7366 • pennmedicine.org/cancer

Case Comprehensive Cancer Center/
University Hospitals Seidman Cancer
Center and Cleveland Clinic Taussig
Cancer Institute
Cleveland, Ohio
800.641.2422 • UH Seidman Cancer Center
uhhospitals.org/services/cancer-services
866.223.8100 • CC Taussig Cancer Institute
my.clevelandclinic.org/departments/cancer
216.844.8797 • Case CCC
case.edu/cancer

City of Hope National Medical Center
Duarte, California
800.826.4673 • cityofhope.org

Dana-Farber/Brigham and Women's
Cancer Center | Massachusetts General
Hospital Cancer Center
Boston, Massachusetts
617.732.5500 • youhaveus.org
617.726.5130
massgeneral.org/cancer-center

Duke Cancer Institute
Durham, North Carolina
888.275.3853 • dukecancerinstitute.org

Fox Chase Cancer Center
Philadelphia, Pennsylvania
888.369.2427 • foxchase.org

Fred & Pamela Buffett Cancer Center
Omaha, Nebraska
402.559.5600 • unmc.edu/cancercenter

Fred Hutchinson Cancer
Research Center/Seattle
Cancer Care Alliance
Seattle, Washington
206.606.7222 • seattlecca.org
206.667.5000 • fredhutch.org

Huntsman Cancer Institute
at the University of Utah
Salt Lake City, Utah
800.824.2073 • huntsmancancer.org

Indiana University
Melvin and Bren Simon
Comprehensive Cancer Center
Indianapolis, Indiana
888.600.4822 • www.cancer.iu.edu

Mayo Clinic Cancer Center
Phoenix/Scottsdale, Arizona
Jacksonville, Florida
Rochester, Minnesota
480.301.8000 • Arizona
904.953.0853 • Florida
507.538.3270 • Minnesota
mayoclinic.org/cancercenter

Memorial Sloan Kettering
Cancer Center
New York, New York
800.525.2225 • mskcc.org

Moffitt Cancer Center
Tampa, Florida
888.663.3488 • moffitt.org

O'Neal Comprehensive
Cancer Center at UAB
Birmingham, Alabama
800.822.0933 • uab.edu/onealcancercenter

Robert H. Lurie Comprehensive Cancer
Center of Northwestern University
Chicago, Illinois
866.587.4322 • cancer.northwestern.edu

Roswell Park Comprehensive
Cancer Center
Buffalo, New York
877.275.7724 • roswellpark.org

Siteman Cancer Center at Barnes-
Jewish Hospital and Washington
University School of Medicine
St. Louis, Missouri
800.600.3606 • siteman.wustl.edu

St. Jude Children's
Research Hospital/
The University of Tennessee
Health Science Center
Memphis, Tennessee
866.278.5833 • stjude.org
901.448.5500 • uthsc.edu

Stanford Cancer Institute
Stanford, California
877.668.7535 • cancer.stanford.edu

The Ohio State University
Comprehensive Cancer Center -
James Cancer Hospital and
Solove Research Institute
Columbus, Ohio
800.293.5066 • cancer.osu.edu

The Sidney Kimmel Comprehensive
Cancer Center at Johns Hopkins
Baltimore, Maryland
410.955.8964
www.hopkinskimmelcancercenter.org

The University of Texas
MD Anderson Cancer Center
Houston, Texas
844.269.5922 • mdanderson.org

UC Davis
Comprehensive Cancer Center
Sacramento, California
916.734.5959 • 800.770.9261
health.ucdavis.edu/cancer

UC San Diego Moores Cancer Center
La Jolla, California
858.822.6100 • cancer.ucsd.edu

UCLA Jonsson
Comprehensive Cancer Center
Los Angeles, California
310.825.5268 • cancer.ucla.edu

UCSF Helen Diller Family
Comprehensive Cancer Center
San Francisco, California
800.689.8273 • cancer.ucsf.edu

University of Colorado Cancer Center
Aurora, Colorado
720.848.0300 • coloradocancercenter.org

University of Michigan
Rogel Cancer Center
Ann Arbor, Michigan
800.865.1125 • rogelcancercenter.org

University of Wisconsin
Carbone Cancer Center
Madison, Wisconsin
608.265.1700 • uwhealth.org/cancer

UT Southwestern Simmons
Comprehensive Cancer Center
Dallas, Texas
214.648.3111 • utsouthwestern.edu/simmons

Vanderbilt-Ingram Cancer Center
Nashville, Tennessee
877.936.8422 • vicc.org

Yale Cancer Center/
Smilow Cancer Hospital
New Haven, Connecticut
855.4.SMILOW • yalecancercenter.org

Index

Made in United States
Troutdale, OR
03/15/2024

18492773R00031